Healthier, Happier
And Well!

Aries Ford

BS, RDN, LDN

Table of contents

DEDICATION

This book is dedicated to increasing wellness education and lifestyle changes as well as empowering individuals to reclaim their health throughout the life cycle.

ACKNOWLEDGMENTS

To my family and friends who have supported me as a dietitian.

Introduction

I promise you that this book will change your life forever. Enclosed are the keys and strategies to be healthier and to increase your overall quality of life. This book includes information for the entire family. You chose the right book, if you want to eat healthier, be happier and live well. My name is Aries Ford and I am your dietitian. I am here to help you reach your goals and encourage you every step of the way. Let's get started!

Chapter 1

Eating Emotionally

Feast - often thought of as a very large, rich, delightfully, well-prepared abundant meal. Everybody gets excited when they hear the word feast. We think "party time!" Why is it that we always look forward to holidays? Is it that we are anticipating spending time with our immediate family and close relatives, or are we just looking forward to the buffet and our own personal "all you can eat contest?"

Another thought? Are you an emotional eater?

Emotional eating is a disorder. When one feels depressed, sad, incomplete, they eat to fill the hole that is empty within them. Most common foods of choice is as follows: Chocolate, mashed potatoes, popcorn, French fries, ice cream, cake, burritos, trail mix, anything one is craving. (Urban dictionary)

Eating to feed a feeling, and not a growling stomach, is emotional eating, "The types of comfort foods a person is drawn toward varies depending on their mood. People in happy moods tended to prefer foods such as pizza or steak (32%). Sad people reached for ice cream and cookies 39% of the time, and 36% of bored people opened up a bag of potato chips (web MD).

Emotional eating food choices only provide euphoric feelings for a limited amount of time. It doesn't make the feeling go away or solve the problem. It comes right back after you have finished your snack or meal.

Dietitians recommend taking steps to combat emotional eating of comfort foods. The first step is to determine how you feel before you decide to eat certain foods. It helps to keep a food log and also write down your feelings beside your food choices.

Drink a glass of water first and think about how to handle your feelings. Water can also determine whether or not you're really hungry. It's natural to feel as if you are hungry when you are dehydrated. The second step is to avoid eating if you don't feel a physical stomach growl or if you do not have diabetes or hypoglycemia. The third step is to take control of situations you can control and let go of the situations that are out of your control. You've won!

Many people suffer from diabetes, hypertension, cancer, obesity and over 25 million people have diabetes. Over 7 million people don't know they have it and over 79 million people have pre-diabetes (which is the medical term given to those who are on the verge of developing diabetes.) 68 million adults have high blood pressure and are taking blood pressure lowering drugs. 71 million people have bad cholesterol levels and more than 35% of the people in the United States are obese. Health risks are determined by using your weight and height to calculate a number called the body mass index (BMI). BMI under 18.5 = (underweight) and 18.5 - 24.9 = (healthy weight) and 25 - 29.9 = (overweight) and 30 or higher = (obese).

You can also use the waist to hip ratio to determine your risk especially for men with an abundance of muscle that is very active in sports. The BMI chart does not take into account muscle mass. Waist circumference is a good indicator of abdominal fat which is a predictor of risk for obesity related diseases. Overweight and obesity is caused by eating too many calories and inactivity. Health consequences include diabetes, coronary heart disease, cancer, high blood pressure, high lipid levels, stroke, liver and gallbladder disease, sleep apnea, osteoarthritis and gynecological problems. The initial treatment should be dietary changes. In other words, changing what we put in our mouths and how often we bend that elbow.

Health can be defined as the state of complete physical, mental and social well-being or the condition of being sound in body, mind and spirit. Healthy doesn't mean you have to weigh 100 lbs! Healthy can be losing 20 lbs if you are overweight (BMI > 25) or gaining 20 lbs if you are under weight (BMI < 18). I have counseled people and have seen the affects of losing even 10% or gaining 10%. I've seen huge improvements in lab values (blood work) and some people were able to lower their dose of medications or gained the ability to stop their meds with doctor's approval. What kinds of changes do we need to make? Activity and physical changes in eating and activity habits. I have counseled people for years as a dietitian and have seen the best results with individuals who allowed themselves to let go of stress and from whatever it is that is hindering them from their health goals. Sometimes past mindsets, pain or loneliness can hinder us. One of the biggest hindrances that people express is fear. There are many sources of fear. Some forms of fear or other hindrances can come from something that happened during childhood or maybe something was said during your childhood. It can be anything. It can simply be that you had very little to eat and developed a habit of eating everything on your plate when you were served a meal or it could be the feeling of not being loved. Another example can be related to poor education regarding healthy food choices and exercise or just not enough time. Hindrances can be stress related or just pure laziness. Hey, we all get lazy and procrastinate at times. Now that you've recognized it, the rest is easy. Success is waiting for you. Read on and read about how an individual counseled is on her way to success.

1. I met with a woman who loved to read books, but she was still hurting inside. She would eat through her loneliness and stressful days. She wanted to lose weight but couldn't because she had difficulty laying her burdens down. She wasn't going to show up to our appointment, but her husband encouraged her to come to

the consultation. She didn't know she was actually meeting me for some extra encouragement. She wanted to lose the amount of weight needed to be healthy again. She was taking over 20 medications to alleviate the symptoms of various diseases. She was simply miserable and tired of the way she was feeling. She was tired of people starring at her. All she needed was a little strength to move forward in her weight loss Strength to fill the void other using food to fill the void. During our session she was able to lift the burdens and heal her heart.

Focus, determination and strength is going to set the foundation of getting our individual and physical bodies in shape. We need to be in unity before we go any further. I need you to say out loud "I am ready to get in shape!" Let's get started! You can do it!

Chapter 2

Eating Intelligently

1- Don't drink your calories! Drink water or unsweetened drinks only. Americans spend an estimated $14.3 billion dollars on sugary drinks. Did you know that dehydration triggers memory loss? We will start to forget if we don't consume enough water. Symptoms of dehydration include: confusion, dizziness, dry skin, dry mouth, fatigue, thirst, headache and constipation. Dark colored urine indicates dehydration. Light colored urine indicates good hydration. Mild to moderate dehydration can be treated with re-hydration (drinking water infused with electrolytes).   Severe dehydration may require medical attention.

Water also helps to jump start your metabolism and is required in for various functions at the cellular level.

Most people simply don't consume enough water. Our bodies need at least 6 to 8 glasses of water a day. Sweetened drinks have a quick impact on your blood sugar levels and provide you with lots of empty calories that can cause you to gain weight. A can of soda can have as much calories as a glazed doughnut. I've seen people lose 1 to 2 pounds a week just by stopping regular sodas.

2- Don't skip meals! What do we do when we skip a meal? We inhale the entire kitchen table the next time we sit down to eat. This causes us to take in extra calories that will cause weight gain. Instead, try to have a small healthy snack if you are unable to eat within a reasonable time frame.

3- Think balance. Eat a variety of foods at meal time. Don't eat an entire plate of mac-n-cheese for dinner. Be sure to include meat or vegetable protein, starch, vegetables and fruit for dessert. Your body requires a variety of foods to provide vital nutrients to jump start metabolism and initiate other functions at the cellular level.

4- Watch those portions! The plate method is the easiest way to watch portions. No, you cannot pile the plate up like a mountain peak. Half of your plate should be non-starchy vegetables other than beans, corn and potatoes (these are considered starches.) A serving of starch is usually 1/3 to ½ cup serving. You should include 3 oz of meat (which is the size of the palm of your hand) or vegetable protein. Vegetarians are allowed more vegetable proteins or protein substitutes to meet their protein needs. They include beans, nuts, soy, tofu, hummus, peanut butter, almond butter and cheese. A ½ ounce of nuts, 1 tablespoon of peanut butter, ¼ cup of beans or 1 egg is equal to 1 ounce of meat protein. Most people need at least 6 ounces of protein per day. These are general serving guidelines. Please consult a registered dietitian for a personal meal plan and the right serving sizes to meet your individual needs.

5- Balance your carbohydrates (starches such as pasta, rice, bread, beans, potatoes, and corn), fruit, milk and sweets. It's very important that we don't over indulge on these foods. Please contact a registered dietitian or myself if you have diabetes for an individualized meal plan.

6- Watch portions of meat and choose lean meats. 3 oz is a general guideline or the size of the palm of your hand. Choose baked, broiled or grilled meats instead of fried. Watch the cheese. Try adding more vegetable proteins to your meals like peanut butter, nuts and beans instead of meat a few times per week.

7- Eat less fat. Choose lower fat items at restaurants and at the grocery store. Watch servings of salad dressings, butter/margarine, sour cream, cream cheese, cheese, whole milk, and gravies, processed meats (sausage, bacon, and hotdogs.) Choose foods that are baked or grilled. Try rice or almond milk instead of whole milk.

8- Watch the salt. Try not to add salt at the table and reduce processed foods, meats, TV dinners, instant flavored potato/rice boxed mixes and soups. Choose fresh or frozen vegetables most of the time or rinse off the canned vegetables at home.

9- Read food labels and choose lower fat and sodium choices.

10- Try to use other seasonings while cooking instead of salt and butter. Garlic powder, lemon pepper, onion powder and lemon juice are some good substitutions that add flavor. You can also season foods with a variety of vegetables such as colorful peppers and onions.

Chapter 3

Weight loss Ideas and Alcohol

- Eat at least 3 small meals per day.
- Try not to go more than 5 hrs between meals
- Know when you are hungry. A good rule is a stomach growl.
- Drink a glass of water before each meal and drink water during your meals.
- Don't eat in front of the TV. Your stomach sends the signal to the brain that you are full, but your brain is occupied watching TV which increases your chances of over eating.
- Use smaller plates and bowls.
- Eat slowly and put your fork or spoon down while you chew. Cut your food one bite at a time.
- Brush your teeth after you eat.
- Cook when you are not hungry and drink water while you cook.
- Be careful of emotional eating- Don't eat because you are bored or sad. Read an

inspirational book, call a friend, listen to music or take a walk.
- Be careful of over indulging in alcohol. I gram of alcohol has almost as much calories as 1 gram of fat. Cocktails, mixed drinks, beer and wine can really pack on the calories. Watch the syrups and sodas added to these drinks. They add extra calories. Alcohol also lowers your blood sugar which can induce hunger and lead to overeating and hypoglycemia.

Consult a dietitian for more details or weight gain tips for underweight individuals.

Chapter 4

What's Your Road Block

Now we can tackle some of the common road blocks since we have the basic tools to support a generally healthy diet. Road blocks are all the excuses we use and know so well. Which one is yours?

1. I am too stress out.
2. Too exhausted.
3. Not enough time to cook.
4. No time to plan and prepare meals.
5. Everybody else is eating it.
6. I haven't eaten all day.
7. I'm upset.
8. Not sure how to read food lables.
9. No time to exercise.
10. Too expensive to eat healthy and the food taste like cardboard.
11. No exercise equipment.
12. I work at a resturant. How do you expect me to eat healthy?
13. I'm too busy.
14. No one to walk with me, and I don't want to leave the house.
15. I have leg problems.
16. No support.
17. I just went to the salon and my hair is beautiful. I can't exercise now.

How to Overcome Your Road Blocks

1. Exercise helps to relieve stress and so does spiritual meditation. Read the bible. Have you ever encountered someone stressed out and angry reading the bible? The bible is one of the quickest stress relievers that I know.
2. We are only human and we all get tired. We never have a problem finding time to do the pleasurable things that we want to do. Find a time during the day that you aren't so tired to exercise. Find time during the week to shop instead of getting fast processed food.
3. Some days are filled with many errands and work and our families. Try cooking one or two days during the week and freezing leftovers for the other days of the week that you don't have time to cook on. Now you can eat healthy, home cooked meals and you don't have to run out and get fast food.
4. You don't have to eat what everyone else is eating at work or family gatherings. You can make healthy choices and you can choose smaller portions.
5. You don't need special exercise equipment to exercise. You can do chair exercises even if you have lower body mobility issues. Simply put small water bottles in your hands and raise your arms in an up and down motion. Your body will still get a work out. Your body was designed to move, not just sit around all day. You will feel better once you get moving.

Chapter 5

How Do I Recognize What Affects How Much I Eat

1. Going to the movies- rent a movie for home and make air popped corn or limit your portions or avoid snacks at the movies.
2. Watching TV with family- don't eat while watching TV. Chew gum.
3. Employee birthday parties- bring a healthy item and watch portion sizes.
4. Vending machines by my office- bring your own healthy snacks from home.
5. Driving in the car passing fast food- make it a rule never to eat in the car.
6. Going shopping hungry- eat a snack before you go and be careful with coupons. Only buy what you need.
7. Neighborhood parties and pot lucks- bring a healthy dish and eat on a small plate.
8. Your spouse or children are eating high fat-high calorie snacks after dinner- keep healthy low fat snacks in the house for yourself.
9. Buffets- try to avoid these if possible. When going out to eat, please choose healthy options from menus, eat a small healthy snack before

going out and drink plenty of water before and during the meal.

  a. Split entrees
  b. Avoid appetizers and desserts or share
  c. Make healthy substitutions
  d. Watch portions
  e. Be firm and remember your goals

10. I'm having a snack attack! - keep bite size veggies and fruits in sight. Leave all the high fat snack foods on the shelf in the grocery store. Try a handful of nuts and raisins to hold you over until your next scheduled meal time.

Chapter 6

Food Safety In My Home

Listed are a few_Basic Food Safety Precautions to keep you and your family safe from harmful food-borne illnesses, food poisoning and bad bacteria.

- Wash hands, counters and utensils thoroughly.
- Use two separate cutting boards for meats and produce.
- Wash produce thoroughly and watch for recalls on contaminated produce
- Disinfect all counter tops before and after food preparation. Especially after raw meats.
- Replace sponges often or wash them in the dishwasher.
- Cook meats until well done.
- Refrigerate food after 2 hours of holding.
- It is best to defrost meats in a sturdy container on the bottom shelf in the fridge instead of on the kitchen counter or sink.
- Always keep cold foods and salads below 40 degrees.
- Good rule of thumb is to keep cold foods cold and hot foods hot!

Chapter 7

Let's Go Shopping For Real

Grocery shopping tips

- Make a list to save time and money. It only makes sense to look at the sales paper to determine what's on sale first. Look in your cabinets and see what you really need from the sale items to start making healthy meals at home. Now you are ready to create a list to provide meals for the next 7 days or so. Consider vegetarian meals during the week as well.

- Start in the produce aisle first. Look for colorful, nutrient rich fruits and vegetables. Bright colors indicate more antioxidants which help to protect the body. Produce is also rich in fiber and very low in calories. Half of your lunch and dinner plate should be filled with selections from the produce aisle. Watch for recalls on contaminated produce.

- Next we can look for dry items and save the cold items for last. We need to keep those items cold as long as possible.

- Shop for whole grain items such as breads, pasta, and rice. Don't forget the nuts and beans.

Now we can shop for lean skinless meats, fish and low fat and fat free dairy. You can also replace your dairy with rice or almond milk and green leafy

Vegetables. Lean meats include skinless chicken and turkey breast, beef cuts without marbling (fat), (sparingly) round steak tenderloin, sirloin tips and center cuts. Don't forget to keep raw meats on the bottom of the cart to prevent cross contamination.

Frozen items should be last in order to keep them frozen as long as possible during travel. You can shop for frozen unbreaded meats/fish, fruits, vegetables, whole grain breakfast items and sorbets. Sometimes frozen foods can be more cost effective, and they are packed with nutrients.

Try not to shop for foods that have a lot of added ingredients such as fat, sugar and salt such as : processed foods, boxed rice, pasta and potato mixes, canned soups, TV dinners, breaded meats and vegetables, bacon, sausage, tuna canned in oil, beans cooked in lard, vegetables cooked in cream or cheese sauces, fried vegetables, sweet rolls, doughnuts, pastries, biscuits, fried tortillas, sugar coated cereals, juices or drinks sweetened with sugar, fruit canned in heavy syrup, 2% or whole milk, regular cheese, yogurt with sugar, hot dogs, and meat with skin.

These foods are high in calories, fat, sodium and or sugar. Moderation is the key as well as finding these choices with reduced sodium, sugar and fat.

Canned foods tend to be high in sodium. Try to purchase reduced sodium or no added salt. You can also rinse your vegetables thoroughly to remove the sodium before consuming. Purchase snacks that are low in fat, sodium, sugar and free of Trans fats or hydrogenated oils. Good snacks include bite size raw fruits and vegetables, unsalted pretzels, animal crackers, Jell-O or pudding. Sherbet and sorbet are good choices. Good snack choices include items that contain less than 5 grams of fat per serving.

How Can I stretch My Meals?

I don't want to leave this page without informing you on how to stretch meals.

- Buy what's on sale
- Buy in bulk
- Freeze leftovers
- Add pasta to soups, stews and chilies to make them more filling
- Replace meat with low cost proteins such as beans and eggs to meals
- Enjoy more casseroles throughout the week

Chapter 8

Food Labels That Count

There are two types of label reading. What to look at when you have time and what to look at when you don't have much time such as during grocery shopping.

Look for these basic label readings at a glance while shopping. Fat and sodium content is the most important items to read on the food label during shopping if you are new at reading labels and want to save time. You can worry about the serving size and carbohydrate count when you get home. Items high in fat will most likely be high in calories. Eating too much fat makes us fat. Healthy eating means reducing the fat and sodium we consume. You also want to be familiar with high fiber choices. Choose food items with greater than 5 grams of fiber per serving.

Don't forget that it is also important to know what's in your food. Let me show you what to look for on a label. Find a label in your kitchen and follow along with me.

Serving size- determines the amount of calories and nutrients in one serving. You have to add more calories if you decide to eat more or the entire package. The same idea goes for fat, sodium and carbohydrates as well.

Fat grams- Compare products and choose foods with the least amount of total fat grams- less than 5 grams of fat per serving for snack foods.

Sodium- Try to choose foods lowest in sodium. 140mg is a good goal per serving.

Carbohydrates- One serving of carbohydrates is equivalent to 15 grams of carbohydrates. A sugar gram is just a component of carbohydrates. Carbohydrates break down into sugar. Seek a dietitian if you want a personalized carbohydrate controlled meal plan.

Fiber- Try to choose items with 5 grams or more per serving.

Chapter 9

Keep On Moving

There are many benefits to physical activity. Dancing to your favorite song like nobody's watching can jump start your weight loss, maintain your weight and prevent further weight gain. Other benefits include:

- Preventing and managing health conditions and disease, strengthen bones to reduce falls, improves heart health, and improves blood sugar and blood pressure levels as well.
- Boost energy levels by delivering more oxygen to your tissues.
- Improves your mood, releases stress and improves confidence. You look better and feel better about yourself.
- Promotes better sleep at night.

Consider at least 30 minutes of daily physical activity. You may need to increase your minutes if your goal is weight loss. Exercising large muscle groups is an effective way to burn fat and gain muscle. Add weight baring exercises to your weekly workouts. One pound weight loss per week is equivalent to burning 3500 calories. That's 500 calories a day or a 16 oz. soda and 3 small cookies per day. You can start slow and build up to 30-60 minutes a day. Some people do 10 minutes three times a day initially. Do what works for you. Stop when you feel abnormally tired and stay hydrated by drinking plenty of water. It is suggested to consult with your physician if you are just starting with exercise for your own safety.

10 Tips to increase your physical activity

1. Post a reminder on the fridge, on the TV and on the bathroom mirror.

2. Put the exercise equipment in front of the TV.

3. Keep your gym shoes in the car or by the front door.

4. Leave an exercise DVD on the coffee table.

5. Hang an activity calendar up at work.

6. Walk on your lunch break.

7. Make a walking date with a friend.

8. Power-walk listening to bible verses.

9. Take the stairs.

10. Park far and walk. Get on the move!

Chapter 10

Staying and Remaining Motivated!

Staying motivated during exercising and eating healthy becomes easier when you don't forget to recognize when you are doing well. Self-monitor, seek support, and add variety to your routines. Keep track of your weight and eating habits with a food record and activity record. If you stumble, that's ok, just get back up and keep trying. Set goals and reward yourself with non-food related activities. It's ok to take a break for a day or two. It's just important not to stop.

Food Record_____

Activity Record_____

My Goals_____

Chapter 11

Vegan, Vegetarian and Flexitarian

Current trends in meatless diets are increasing daily. Millions of Americans are gravitating to vegetarianism. Can this be healthy? Let's take a look at why, but first I want to introduce a few terms.

Vegan- does not eat meat, poultry, seafood, or products containing (gelatin, broth, gravy and lard). Also does not eat eggs or products containing eggs milk, dairy foods (such as cheese, yogurt, ice cream, whey, casein) or honey.

Vegetarian- (Lacto-ovo) - does not eat meat, poultry, seafood, or products containing

(Lacto)- does not eat meat, poultry, seafood, or products containing. Also, does not eat eggs or products containing eggs (such as many baked goods)

Flexitarian- (semi vegetarian) consumes mostly plant based diet but will occasionally eat meat and meat products when they have the urge.

Some of the reasons by individuals choose to follow this trend includes: it's healthier, cost saving for due to food safety concerns.

However, can you eat a balanced meal by eating this type of diet? Can you obtain all the nutrients you need eating this type of diet? Could this be healthy for children?

You can eat balanced as long as you include food servings from all food groups at meal times with adequate amounts of plant proteins. You can obtain all the nutrients you need while eating a balanced plant based diet with the exception of B12. This is a vitamin only found in animal products. Children can maintain health and grow adequately as long as they consume enough plant based proteins to meet their growing needs as well as a B12 supplement. Suggest consulting a dietitian or physician for adequate B12 supplementation. This vitamin is fat soluble and can be dangerous in excessive amounts.

Most people typically don't consume enough protein and most people don't even realize it. Protein is needed to maintain muscle mass and is essential for healthy skin and hair. Vegetable proteins or protein substitutes can meet your protein needs. You can select from a variety of beans, nuts and seeds, soy, tofu, hummus, peanut butter and almond butter. Please take caution if you have a medical condition that does not permit you to consume nuts or seeds. You may seek a dietitian or me for a special consultation. ½ ounce of nuts, 1 tablespoon of peanut butter or other nut butters, 1/2 cup of beans is equal to 1 ounce of meat protein or 7 grams of protein. Most people need at least 6 – 8 ounces of protein per day or 42-56 grams per day. The amount of protein that you need is based on your current body weight. These are general serving guidelines. Please consult a registered dietitian for a personal meal plan and the right serving sizes to meet your individual needs. You can also increase your protein intake by adding brown rice and a high protein breakfast cereal to your meals. ½ cup of brown rice can add as much as 5 grams of protein and a serving of a high protein cereal for breakfast can add as much as 9-15 grams of protein. I would suggest adding at least 2 ounces of protein to all meals and 1-2 ounces of protein with snacks. Protein will help to add balance to your meals and aid in fullness.

7 grams of protein power listed below

1/2 ounce of nuts or 23 almonds

1 tablespoon of peanut butter or other nut butters

1/2 cup of beans

1/2 cup brown rice

High protein cereal (grams of protein and serving size will vary. Read the food label)

Add these to your meal plan. Double up to get the right number of protein grams for the day

Chapter 12

Should I Supplement?

Vitamins and minerals serve vital functions in the human body. They are needed to literally keep us alive and healthy. Your health risk increases if your nutritional needs are not balanced. It is ideal to obtain 100% of our nutrients from food in its natural state. However, this does not always happen. Most individuals are not able to meet all of their nutritional needs by food alone. It helps to balance our nutrients by eating what our body needs to function or by supplementing what's required for normal organ function. Supplements are products intended to supplement our diets. Not to be used as the first choice. For example, some individuals will consume an over the counter fiber supplement instead of increasing fruits and vegetables in their daily meal pattern.

What supplements are safe? There are so many to choose from including but not limited to: vitamins, minerals, weight loss supplements, herbal supplements, electrolyte supplements and protein supplements. There is a possibility of taking too much of a good thing. Here's why. The FDA must be notified of a new supplement on the market. However,

FDA approval of a supplement is not required and not regulated. The FDA will only remove a product if an adverse reaction was reported. Fat soluble vitamins are stored in the liver and can be dangerous in excessive amounts.

What You Should Do Before Supplementing

- Discuss supplementation with your doctor or dietitian.

- Request blood work (labs) from your primary care physician. Labs indicate deficiencies in the human body and will direct your doctor regarding what to supplement and the amount of supplementation.

- Never take more than the recommended amount.

- Never take more than one multivitamin product at the same time unless directed by your doctor to prevent an over dose.

- Talk to your doctor about your current health conditions. You may need a special vitamin with less potassium.

- Talk to your pharmacist regarding your current medications and possible interactions with vitamin and mineral supplements

Your personal checklist of questions:

Chapter 13

Changing the World with Healthier Children

Childhood obesity continues to grow at a ridiculously rate. We must take control and help our children. I met a woman who told me that her son ate so much when she left the house to run errands that she had to pack most of the household food supply in her trunk. This should not be happening. Children are having tantrums for food items. This should not be happening.

What are some of the reasons for childhood obesity, what are the risks and what can we do about it?

Some of the reasons include but not limited to: processed foods/ high fat fast foods, overall lack of nutrition knowledge of parents, working parents who are too tired to cook a healthy meal, children eating alone, families not eating at the table together, stress at school, inactivity and too much screen time.

Risk includes diabetes, high blood pressure, high cholesterol and other obesity related disease issues as well as low self esteem.

What can we do about it? Actually, what must we do about it?

- Establish physical activity early. Daily exercise as a family. Find something that your child enjoys.

- Server a balanced breakfast

- Provide healthy lunches

- Limit sweetened beverages

- Limit eating out

- Instill healthy eating habits beginning in infancy

- Encouraged baked food items instead of fried

- Limit candy and junk food

- Sit down family meals at home

- Limit screen time(TV, games, IPads, smart phones)

- Model healthy eating habits

- Choose to make a lifestyle change.

- Encourage your child to choose something new out of the produce section of the grocery store.

Chapter 14

Aging Gracefully

Have you ever looked at someone after asking their age and wondered why they looked older or younger than the number they gave you? Have you wondered why your old classmates from 20 years ago have aged much faster or slower than you have?

It is important to maintain your health at all ages. There are many concerns for older adults as we age. Your metabolism will begin to slow down and your taste may be altered. Older Americans experience a reduction in the ability to absorb key nutrients, dehydration and a sluggish digestive system. Therefore, it is imperative to consume adequate water, B vitamins, fiber and less fat. It is important to eat less calories if you are overweight and nutrient dense or high calorie foods if you are underweight. Simple walking exercises are suggested to strengthen your heart and bones. Eating nutritionally and exercising are successful keys to a more energized, healthier, younger looking body.

About the Author

"Obtain the Keys, Expect Success and Achieve Breakthrough Results"

Aries Ford, RDN, LDN is a dietitian, motivational speaker specializing in nutrition conferences and workshops. Aries has over 15 years of experience as a dietitian in planning, implementing and coordinating clinical patient nutritional care to promote health and control various diseases. Aries experience includes but not limited to: Nutrition Support Dietitian, extensive knowledge in counseling individuals and providing appropriate interventions of various disease conditions in clinical, community and nursing home environments. Experience also extends in developing curriculum, teaching groups and evaluating training techniques. A graduate of the University of North Carolina at Greensboro and a Buffalo NY native. You may have seen appearances by Aries on WXII 12.

- "Parents balancing work and family" WXII
- "Moms saving Time" WXII
- TCP and Triad Fitness and Health Magazines
- "Inside TV" with Valarie Persaud in New Jersey
- Real Health Real Beauty Radio Show WEAC 860

VISIT MY WEBSITE

ARIESFORD.ORG

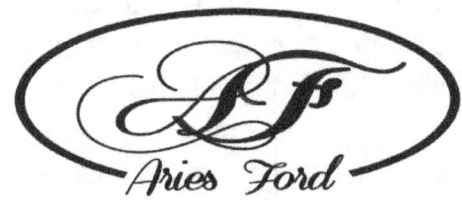

$\mathcal{D}$ISCLAIMER

This book is written to promote nutrition, health and healing. Please seek a professional dietitian before starting a nutrition plan.

Recommended Readings and References

Selections from the Academy of Nutrition and Dietetics and the CDC